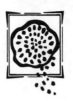

Seeds of Strength

Catholic Thinking on End of Life Decisions

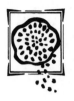

Catholic Thinking on End of Life Decisions

by
Rev. Michael P. Orsi, Ed.D.

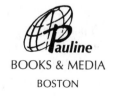

BOOKS & MEDIA

BOSTON

Nihil Obstat:
        Rev. John J. Connelly

Imprimatur:
        †Bernard Cardinal Law
        April 23, 1999

ISBN 0-8198-7025-0

Printed and published in the U.S.A. by Pauline Books & Media, 50 Saint Pauls Avenue, Boston, MA 02130-3491.

www.pauline.org

Pauline Books & Media is the publishing house of the Daughters of St. Paul, an international congregation of women religious serving the Church with the communications media.

1 2 3 4 5 6   05 04 03 02 01 00

*To my father
who lived and died
a Christian gentleman*

Contents

Guidelines for the Sick

"No matter how long we have, we always want a little more," my father said to me on the last morning of his life. Having attained almost 80 years of age, he knew his life was nearing its end. He had been ailing for about 15 years, enduring a variety of illnesses. But his feisty nature, the wonders of modern medical technology, and prayer, helped him to cheat death numerous times. Nevertheless, this *Come-Back Kid,* as we dubbed him, always reminded the family that in the end death must come to everyone.

This very sobering thought could lead a person to three mutually exclusive and unchristian attitudes toward sickness:

a) why bother fighting for life;
b) life should be preserved at all costs;
c) despair of God's love and concern.

Perhaps in the course of an illness you have entertained all three of the above attitudes to some degree. This booklet is designed to give some context to the difficulty of serious or terminal illness (which may be your present situation) and to help individuals and their families to make good decisions regarding treatment and care. The guidelines contained in this booklet are presented in the light of the Christian belief that our bodily life is a God-given good, but not the highest good. It is superseded only by our life with God in heaven which is the highest good or perfection the human person can attain.

Progress has made contemporary living easier in many ways. It has also tended to further complicate the difficult decisions we must sometimes make, particularly in the area of health care and end of life issues. What makes health care decisions so difficult is the ability of modern medicine, with its team approaches, staged surgical techniques, monitoring capabilities, and ventilatory support systems, to keep almost anyone technically alive. This has gradually shifted the problem in question from having the means to reverse the dying process to that of measuring the quality of life sustained and preserved. Given the power and capacity that these new technologies provide, we have the corresponding responsibility of making good health care judgments based on our Judeo-Christian beliefs.

Dealing with Your Feelings

Perhaps the best way to proceed is to first of all deal honestly with our feelings about sickness and death. No one likes to feel sick. No one wants to die. Yet, due to the effects of Original Sin, everyone must eventually succumb to natural bodily breakdown. When faced with the absolute reality of death, all of us must deal with seven basic and very natural emotions or reactions, sometimes simultaneously:

- Fear of pain and the uncertainty of the grave;
- Anger over why this is happening;
- Bargaining: I will lead a better life if my illness can be beat;
- Denial of the illness;
- Depression leading one into isolation;
- Acceptance of death if it is God's will;
- Detachment from life; tying up loose ends in this world and preparing for the next.

Illness is a time of crisis, but it is also a moment of grace for those who are sick and for those who care for them. Those who suffer illness have the opportunity to be closely configured to Christ's suffering, death and resurrection.

The Paschal Mystery

God joined himself to the human family in the person of Jesus and so we can be certain that he understands our human condition and feelings. By searching the Scriptures we discover a Jesus who wants to heal those who are ill, who weeps at the death of his friend Lazarus, who agonizes over the suffering and death that awaits him on Calvary. In effect, the agony in the garden of Gethsemane was a condensed version of the stages of dying and death that confronted the humanity of Jesus over the course of his public ministry. "Father, let this cup pass if it be your will; though not my will but yours be done" (cf. Mt 26:39). This acceptance of the Father's plan was the critical moment leading to Jesus' suffering, death and resurrection—and our hope for eternal life. Our faith in Christ, which assures us of eternal life, strengthens us to face our present struggles with courage and, in the words of Jesus, to "be not afraid" (cf. Mt 28:10).

Stewardship

Our Judeo-Christian tradition walks a middle path between medical vitalism, which seeks to preserve life at any cost, and medical pessimism, which seeks to kill when life seems frustrating, burdensome, or useless. And the key to this middle way is the foundational belief in the dignity of every human person as made in God's image. The commitment to what human dignity demands for health care and the preservation of life is guided by a common theme of "stewardship." Stewardship implies a personal responsibility to care for the God-given gift of our life. Proper stewardship also means recognizing how and when to let go of that gift by allowing it to take its natural course. Because of the uniqueness of each individual and of particular circumstances, there are very few hard and fast, set-in-stone rules. However, there are some guidelines.

Discernment

Any important medical decision should be, first of all, the fruit of a discernment entered into with a spirit of prayer. Read Sacred Scripture, especially the gospel passages of Jesus' healing miracles and the passion and resurrection accounts. These will lend strength and bring the loving presence of God closer during a time of crisis. Through God's Word we come to perceive more clearly that his plan for us continues to unfold even through sickness. Secondly, seek the guidance and support of a pastor or parish priest. The sacramental ministry of the priest is invaluable during a time of serious illness. The Sacrament of the Sick, of Reconciliation and of the Eucharist, are all vital to any program for physical and spiritual wellness. In light of the effectiveness of prayer for healing, it is wise to engage the prayer support of family, friends and parish family. Thirdly, for any technical concerns encountered in regard to religious obligations or recommended therapies and procedures, turn to Church documents* and professionals who can walk you through them. A good place to start with is your diocesan Chancery office. And lastly, a beneficial approach to any health care decisions that must be made always engages the individual who is ill, their family, doctor and pastor.

Proportionate and Disproportionate Means for Preserving Life

Over the years a basic consideration for preserving life rested with two terms, "ordinary" and "extraordinary" or, in contemporary parlance, "proportionate" and "disproportionate" means. The Catholic Church considers extraordinary (disproportionate) means as "optional," while ordinary means are "obligatory." No one is obliged to do what is extraor-

---

*Pages 56–57.

dinary to prolong their life. That decision belongs to the individual patient or to his or her delegated "health care proxy."

The distinction between ordinary (proportionate) and extraordinary (disproportionate) actions or omissions clusters on three points: first, a treatment, operation, procedure or drug should offer an individual reasonable hope of benefit; second, the medical action should be without serious danger of death; and finally, it should be without excessive pain, hardship, burden, expense or subjective repugnance. If a medical action satisfies all three of the above criteria, then it is ordinary means, while anything which goes beyond these criteria may be deemed extraordinary means by an individual. There is no "check list" of extraordinary measures. Only the above principles or criteria are the stable factors which can be applied in specific, individual cases. You will find the case studies below helpful for understanding how the principles are applied in making a health care decision.

The term *proportionate means,* as used in moral theology, includes all medicines, treatments and operations offering a reasonable hope of benefit for the patient and which can be obtained without excessive expense, pain, or other burdens. *Disproportionate means* refers to all medicines, treatments and operations which cannot be obtained without excessive expense, pain or other burden. When determining whether a particular medicine, procedure or mechanical device is proportionate or disproportionate, one must consider all the relevant circumstances of the case in its clinical and personal dimensions: the condition of the patient, special and familial situations, persons, places, times and culture. Age, medical condition, as well as the imminence of death, also factor into a decision. It is critical to judge each case individually and to also keep in mind whether the treatment is for a dying or non-dying person.

While one may decide to forego disproportionate means to begin with, one may also cease life-saving attempts once the already initiated means are later determined to be disproportionate. Hence treatments begun, by whatever means, can be terminated. Dialysis, for example, may be discontinued as the circumstances of the patient change.

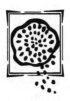

Quality of Life

The key to good stewardship over the gift of life is our ability to recognize it as truly a means for fulfilling our purpose and ultimate goal of being with God. For a Christian, the quality of all life is seen as the most excellent when it is directed toward God. Although the term "quality of life" has nothing to do with a "measuring rod" for determining human excellence, nevertheless, by its very nature, it is somewhat relative, pertaining to the physical, emotional and spiritual state of an individual. Therefore, where an individual may be on their spiritual journey could very well determine the wisest course of action regarding the choices medical care offers. Again, this does not mean there are no guidelines. The Church has established the terms proportionate and disproportionate means to assist individuals in determining what should be done in order to be good stewards of life and to grow in holiness.

With these terms as a guide, perhaps more light can be shed on how to choose what is right for you in your unique situation by presenting real cases of people who worked through important medical decisions. Their stories illustrate proportionate and disproportionate means and will be helpful for understanding the Church's teaching and how to apply it in your particular need.

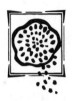

Case Studies

Rose

Disproportionate Means and Comfort Measures Only

A woman of about 50, Rose was married and had two married children. Rose dedicated her life to her family and worked as a homemaker. She involved herself in the life of her parish and generously contributed her time and talents to various local activities.

Generally a healthy woman, Rose began to suffer severe headaches over a period of a few months. She passed it all off as stress. Eventually even the megadoses of aspirin she took no longer relieved her pain. The first sign that something could be seriously wrong began with Rose's experience of double vision. At this point Rose made an appointment to see her doctor.

Medical specialists ran a series of tests and discovered a malignant tumor. In the presence of her husband, children and their parish priest, the doctors told Rose her condition was terminal and then proceeded to present two options for treatment. They could try to operate and thereby extend her life for perhaps a year. The quality of her life, however, would be poor and she would experience a great deal of pain and sickness. Or the doctors could simply allow nature to take its course and provide the care of "comfort measures only." This would mean food, hydration, cleanliness, and palliative care. In this second scenario Rose would gradually lose her faculties of speech, sight, hearing, sensation, etc., but she would also die practically pain-free.

Her family assured her that they would support her one hundred percent in whatever she chose to do without any worry about care or cost. Her parish priest affirmed that in either choice her decision would be in accord with Church teaching.

Rose decided to return home and die peacefully. She felt that her life was coming to its natural conclusion and she would much rather spend the remaining time with her family than in a hospital or nursing home. She did not wish for any extraordinary actions to preserve her life.

During the next six months a hospice nurse visited Rose who received daily care from her family and a home health-care aide. The parish priest's frequent visits to the home were a great spiritual support for Rose and her family. As Rose's illness progressed she slipped into a coma. She passed away peacefully.

By her life and death Rose gave witness to her faith in the Paschal Mystery. Those who knew Rose attested to the fact that she spent the first six months of her illness as real quality time in preparation for her meeting with God. Rose offered her suffering's to God for the souls in purgatory. In many ways the family realized that those months were an exceptional moment of grace for her and them. They often prayed the rosary with Rose, were present during the priest's visits with Viaticum (the Eucharist), and tended to her needs in charity.

An operation would have been the cause of undo burden in Rose's case and disproportionate to the benefit she would have received since it offered no reasonable hope. The few months of life she might have gained would have been filled with excessive pain, hardship, burden and expense for her and her family. The futility of the operation and the subsequent pain could also have proven disruptive to Rose's spiritual life as she prepared for her return to God. Rose made the best choice for herself and her family.

Al

Proportionate Means

Al is a 65-year-old retired police officer. He has three children who live a distance away from him. Al and his wife always planned to travel and visit their family after his retirement, but his wife died suddenly. Then Al's world seemed to fall apart. His wife had always taken care of their social activities and without her Al began losing many of his social contacts. He even began to lose touch with his children.

When one of his daughters arrived for a visit, she immediately noticed Al's right eye bulging out of its socket. She struggled to convince him that he needed to make an appointment with an opthamologist. He finally agreed. Following a number of tests the doctor diagnosed Al as having a benign tumor that was operable. He felt confident that Al had an excellent chance of full recovery. However, without treatment, the tumor could cause very serious complications and eventually lead to disability and death.

Depressed over the loss of his wife and having isolated himself for some time, Al saw no reason to live. He refused treatment saying he wanted to die. He claimed it was his right. (Mental health professionals recommend that major life decisions be avoided while one is in a state of depression. Under its influence people can make bad decisions which they might not make otherwise. Often this has been the case with those who have sought physician assisted suicide. Studies show that individuals who receive proper counseling, and appropriate medications when necessary, usually make a choice for life.)

Al's daughter brought him home from the doctor's office and telephoned her two brothers. When they were all gathered at his home, Al's children began to argue and to try to reason with their father. They could not agree with his refusal to accept treatment. They expressed love and concern for their father, as well as their frustration over his attitude. One of his sons warned Al that his failure to seek medical help could be a sin against the stewardship God had given him over his body; that this refusal was really suicidal. The operation was really quite ordinary. Not only did it promise a high degree of success, but it offered reasonable hope for benefit without excessive burden. Al possessed the necessary financial resources for his medical needs and his children assured him that they would care for him during his recovery. Al truly had an obligation to accept this proportionate means of treatment.

Ultimately, the winning words which changed Al's mind were that his children would care for him after the surgery. Al is now doing well and enjoying life. He keeps in touch with his children and grandchildren who bring him much joy. Proving again that love goes a long way toward healing and giving a person the desire to live.

Mamie

Do Not Resuscitate (DNR)

Mamie was a 92-year-old woman who had lived a very full life and continued to love and enjoy her family. Due to a serious heart condition she had spent the last 10 years living with her daughter. Osteoporosis had also caused her to become so fragile she had already suffered several broken bones. For the most part Mamie was bedridden. Because of her very poor physical condition, bypass or transplant surgeries were not options for treating her severely damaged heart. High medical costs became another factor when considering the low success rate and benefit of such treatment for someone her age. No options were advisable aside from the nitroglycerin tablets Mamie took when she felt extreme pain.

On a particularly painful night, Mamie had great difficulty breathing. Her daughter called for paramedics. They arrived and quickly diagnosed her condition as heart failure. On the way to the hospital Mamie stopped breathing. The emergency medical technicians (EMT's) resuscitated her and by the time they reached the hospital she was breathing again.

Mamie was placed on a respirator immediately. During the next three days her heart stopped four times and each time she was resuscitated. Finally the doctors met with Mamie's daughter. In their conversation with her the doctors indicated there was little hope for her mother's survival. They asked if she would be willing to sign a *Do Not Resuscitate (DNR)* order; the next time her mother's heart stopped beating they would allow her to die peacefully.

Years before, when Mamie's health began deteriorating, she had designated her daughter as her health care proxy. This authorized her to act on her mother's behalf and they had thouroughly discussed Mamie's end of life wishes. Because of the futility of continuing the present procedures, and knowing well that her mother would not want to be kept alive under such circumstances, Mamie's daughter agreed to the DNR order. A day later Mamie died peacefully.

Mamie's full life, the little hope for her recovery as well as the pain and isolation life on a respirator meant, certainly canceled the need for any further heroic effort to preserve her life. Mamie's age, medical condition, and her imminent death were all strong factors in the decision to forgo further life saving attempts. In Mamie's case such attempts had truly become disproportionate means.

Herman

A Feeding Tube Is Not Disproportionate for Those in a Persistent Vegetative State (PVS)

Herman, a energetic young man of 19, was driving his girlfriend to the movies one night when they were hit broadside by a truck. His girlfriend died instantly. Barely alive himself, Herman was flown to a trauma unit by helicopter. At the hospital doctors put Herman on a respirator and performed emergency surgery in an attempt to save his life. Herman was in critical condition and as far as the doctors could determine, would probably remain in a *Persistent Vegetative State (PVS)*.

Days passed with little improvement. Nevertheless, Herman's mother visited him twice a day, leaving her other five children in the care of a trusted friend. She did not give up hope. Every day at the hospital she bathed Herman, brushed his teeth and combed his hair. Some hospital staff members hinted that she was wasting her time since these activities were all part of routine care—and Herman wasn't aware of her presence.

On the twenty-fifth day the doctors determined that Herman's progress was sufficient for him to be taken off the respirator. Assessing that Herman would continue in a Persistent Vegetative State (PVS), the hospital made plans for him to be moved to a long-term nursing care facility. When a few members of the staff suggested that perhaps Herman's feeding tube should also be removed, his mother balked. This would certainly cause him to die of starvation. She knew that such an act contradicted the teaching of the Catholic Church which considers *intubation* (feeding with a tube) an ordinary means of preserving life, especially in a case like Herman's where he was not dying from any pathology. Her son was young and strong and always had a love for life. And besides, she wasn't ready to give up on him.

Then, on the twenty-eighth day, Herman suddenly opened his eyes. He began speaking again and each day made gradual, steady progress. Not too long after regaining consciousness, he was sent to a rehabilitation center where he spent nine months.

Although Herman now has mild brain damage which makes it difficult for him to read and has slurred his speech, he is able to hold a part-time job, drives a truck, and weight-lifts. He was the fourth runner-up in the *Mr. New Jersey Body Building Competition*.

Herman's mother never gave up. Her strength, faith and hope literally helped to save his life. She understood that the quality of Herman's life could not be judged merely on an arbitrary scale based on consciousness and motor skills. A person who is not conscious does not become less human. The very use of the term, "vegetative state," therefore comes into question. It implies that the unconscious individual exists only as a vegetable, incapable of enjoying a human and personal life. Life is a good for a human person as a bodily being, not simply as a conscious subject. Ordinary care that keeps a person alive, no matter what their condition may be, truly benefits that person even if in only a small way. Hydration and nutrition are not judged futile because they fail to achieve a complete recovery from a symptom, pathology or condition which is extrinsic to the need for nutrients.[1] A genuine solidarity of the helpless patient and the caregiver evinces the true dignity of the human person and quality of life; it can be a moment of grace that enhances the caregiver's quality of life too! The moral here is, "Always err on the side of life."

Bob

When the Respirator May Be Removed

Bob was a 68-year-old married man whose four children were grown and married. Diagnosed with cancer of the esophagus which had already metastasized to other parts of his body, the doctors gave him little hope. Nevertheless, they performed sur-

---

1. Cf. Grisez, G. *The Way of the Lord: Living a Christian Life,* vol. II (1993, Quincy, IL) p. 525.

gery to help him in swallowing and to relieve his discomfort.

After the surgery Bob returned home where his wife cared for him. One day as she helped him to eat, a piece of food became lodged in his throat and he began choking. By the time an emergency squad arrived Bob was no longer breathing; oxygen had ceased reaching his brain. The paramedics resuscitated him en route to the emergency room and when they arrived, doctors placed him on a respirator. As the medical team continued with emergency procedures, an electroencephalogram (EEG) revealed that Bob's lower brain waves had ceased. He was now only being kept alive by the respirator.

A representative of the hospital's ethics committee met with Bob's wife and children to explain the situation and to suggest that the respirator be disconnected. Bob was brain-dead and prolonging his life with heroic measures (disproportionate means) was futile. Bob's family agreed. They stood by Bob's bed and said their good-byes. The respirator was disconnected and Bob died within a few hours.

Because Bob was brain-dead his breathing continued only through the power of technological means. No treatment could offer hope or benefit for someone in his medical condition. There were no valid reasons for continuing to fend off his natural death by the use of such procedures. In fact, in this case it would be wrong.

Marion

Palliative Care

Marion, a widow with three married children, was 70 years old and suffering from terminal cancer. Because her doctors held little hope for remission, Marion and her family decided that *comfort measures only* would be the best course to take for her care.

The doctors suggested that Marion be enrolled in a hospice program which would assist with nursing care needs including hygiene and palliative care (pain management). Everyone expected that Marion's cancer would be painful, but the doctors assured Marion and her family that all her pain could be managed. They were also very frank, indicating that some danger did exist that her drug therapy could hasten death. Still, the intention of easing Marion's pain outweighed any danger of shortening her life which was already slowly ebbing away. This decision posed no ethical or moral problems for anyone involved.

After only a few months, Marion quietly slipped into a coma and died peacefully in her sleep.

Palliative care is used to help a person tolerate the pain which accompanies terminal illness. Extreme suffering can prevent a person from preparing spiritually for their death and may lead to despair. So long as the drug therapy used is intended to relieve pain and not to hasten death or kill, palliative care may be used even if the shortening of a person's life also results.

Julia

Removing the Feeding Tube

Julia was a 50-year-old woman who had suffered with emphysema for a number of years. Eventually her condition demanded that she be put on a respirator. She became so weakened that a feeding tube was inserted to provide nourishment.

Julia lapsed into a coma. Sometime later her doctors determined that the feeding tube served only to prolong her natural death. The hospital ethics committee consulted with Julia's family and together they decided to remove the feeding tube. Within days Julia died of her illness, not of induced starvation.

As a person's medical situation changes, new determinations must be made as to what measures should now be taken regarding treatment. Initially Julia's condition required a ventilator and feeding tube. As her condition steadily deteriorated these became disproportionate means. In her case the continuation of feeding with a tube could bring Julia no benefit.

Although feeding and hydration are usually considered proportionate means of preserving life, when a person is dying of a disease and a feeding tube only prolongs their agony and natural death, it may be removed.

Pompeo

Comfort Measures Only

I began this booklet quoting words spoken by my father on the day he died. Let me tell you a little bit more about him and about his death.

For the three years prior to his death Dad was on kidney dialysis. He really did quite well and although it was burdensome, he had a desire to live. During those three years he continued to enjoy his wife, children and grandchildren. He ate well, remained as active as possible for his condition and enjoyed his music, playing the clarinet, mandolin and flute. Dad knew that he could morally stop the dialysis at anytime because in his case it was a disproportionate means.

Three months before his death, Dad noticed his toes were turning black. The vascular surgeons who examined him informed my father that they could do nothing short of amputation because of the severity of the vascular disease. Such an option was inconceivable for Dad. Always an active man, he knew he would not be able to live with the dialysis and disability. Aware that his days were numbered, Dad decided that he would rather go home and spend the remaining time with his family. The doctors provided him with a visiting nurse and palliative care.

Dad's situation fits under the area of the second principle above where a person's repugnance for a particular procedure causes that procedure to be considered disproportionate, and therefore becomes valid grounds for refusal.

As Dad's condition worsened over the last three months of his life, he also developed heart failure which required that he return to the hospital many times. The hospital social workers provided him with a Do Not Resuscitate (DNR) form, which he signed.

I was at home with my father the night before he died. He was experiencing chest pains and severe pain in his legs. My mother and I provided him with prescribed pain killers and care. Dad kept apologizing to us for the trouble he felt he was causing. Sitting next to him on the bed, I assured him that it was no trouble at all, rather, it was a privilege to be able to help him who had always been and done so much for us. Throwing his arm around my neck and drawing me close, he kissed me and said how much he loved me. That will forever be one of my life's most cherished moments. In that instant Christ's humanity, his suffering and his love become more real for me than it had ever been before. Caring for the sick and being loved by the sick is indeed sacramental.

Early in the morning I accompanied Dad on his last trip to the hospital. He spoke at length about his past life uttering "Thank God" with each breath. Grateful for the life God had given him, Dad saw everything as a blessing. His words were truly a hymn of gratitude and praise which deeply touched me. Dad's final conversation really proved to be a summation and testimony to his faith. He was neatly wrapping things up.

I left Dad about 8:00 P.M. that evening, and at about 11:00 P.M. I received a call from the hospital.

Dad's difficulty in breathing had become acute and the doctors wanted to put him on a respirator, but he had refused! I arrived at the hospital within a half-hour and began the ritual, *The Commendation of the Dying.* Dad was ready to meet God. As he breathed his last, it was not a gasp of agony but a sigh of deep thanks to God for his life.

Dad's inner strength and great faith made his final days truly blessed quality time. He made wise end of life decisions and died with the same dignity he had maintained throughout his life. Although illness was difficult for Dad to live with, it was also a time of grace.

The Mass of Christian Burial was a beautiful celebration of thanksgiving for Dad's life in Christ, a life he lived so well. Neither he nor my family had any regrets. We certainly miss him, but our faith assures us that life is not ended but changed. We look forward to being with Dad again in heaven.

Summary

As we have seen, the health care decisions made in each of the cases, relied on the particular circumstances of the person who was ill. Each of these individuals and their families faced one or more of the difficult questions which may arise in making end of life decisions. These examples serve as illustrations of the Church's guidelines and as helps in making your own end of life decisions. Because every case is entirely unique, it is always recommended that you consult with health care professionals, clergy, family and trusted friends as to what options are best for you.

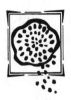

The Living Will

The *Living Will* is a document that provides instructions regarding your medical treatment and care should you be unable to communicate your informed consent because of illness or injury. It is strongly recommended that you have a Living Will. This document is indispensable for your benefit, peace of mind, and the good conscience of those who are close to you. The Living Will may be drawn up by an attorney or a standard form may be provided by your doctor, case worker, hospice representative or your local Catholic hospital or diocesan office. You should sign your Living Will in the presence of two witnesses and acknowledge it in the presence of a notary public.

As a Catholic, your Living Will should contain a presumption in favor of life and provide for necessary medical care and treatment including food and water by mechanical or artificial means if this should be necessary. You should ask that maximum efforts be used to relieve pain, even if shortening your life is an unintended side effect. If you are pregnant, you should include that maximum effort be made to save your life and that of your child.

As Herman's case exemplified, *quality of life* determinations are arbitrary and dangerous. Quality of life decisions can reduce the human person to being thought of in a less than human way. Such an attitude can lead to the cessation of medical treatment and cutting off of food and water, thus inducing death. Be careful not to sign any document which gives another person the unlimited authority to stop your medical treatment and care even when your death is not immanent. Also, bear in mind that no written document can substitute for a competent and moral physician who is faithful to the Hippocratic ethic and tradition.

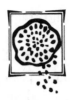

Health Care Proxy
(Durable Power of Attorney)

At the same time you make your Living Will, it is strongly recommended that you appoint a *Health Care Proxy* who will make sure your wishes are carried out. A Health Care Proxy acts on your behalf when you are unable to communicate your informed consent in matters of medical treatment and decisions. Be certain to appoint someone you trust. Your Health Care Proxy should know your mind on issues pertinent to your condition, your moral stance concerning proportionate and disproportionate means of preserving life and end of life issues. A thorough discussion of the above should take place with your designated Health Care Proxy. Be as specific as possible; it will make things much easier for everyone involved. Also be sure to discuss your wishes with your physician. Give copies of your Living Will to your Health Care Proxy, physician and attorney.

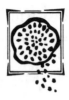

Conclusion

Although illness is a difficult time for an individual as well as their family, it is a natural part of life. This booklet began with the encouraging words "Do Not Be Afraid," and we repeat, *do not be afraid* even in this time of difficulty. As in all moments of life, God's grace has a way of shining through difficulties. The cross of Christ is certainly a prime example of how grace is present in suffering: "Christ, through his own salvific suffering, is very much present in every human suffering.... It is suffering, more than anything else, which clears the way for the grace which transforms human souls."[2]

---

2. Pope John Paul II, *Salvifici Doloris* (Pauline Books & Media, Boston, MA) pp. 45–47.

Only through Jesus' passion could the resurrection occur. Amazing Grace! Perhaps your illness is the cross that leads to your Easter Sunday. In John's Gospel Jesus declares that all who believe will have eternal life when he "is lifted up from the earth" (cf. Jn 3:14–16). The human race is saved at the moment when Christ freely chooses his crucifixion and death. Like Christ, the testimony of your faith in times of suffering and illness will be a grace for you and others. Allow others to share in your suffering; even in serious illness we can be Christ's instruments, evangelizing others to the message of the Gospel of Life.

Those who suffer are united to Christ in a particular way. And those who are united to him in suffering will also share the glory of his resurrection: "For through faith the cross reaches man together with the resurrection."[3] God does not abandon the son or daughter that you became at baptism. Never! Remember the words of Jesus, "I am with you always" (cf. Mt 28:20). For those who drink the cup of suffering that he drank, there is the fulfillment of his promise of the Kingdom of Heaven.

---

3. Ibid, p. 32.

When we take up the cross according to God's will and not our own, it makes each breath of our life, especially the last, a hymn of thanks to him. May your personal Gethsemane open your heart to the Father's will and to the truth of his love for you.

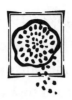

Prayers for the Sick

In times of suffering and illness it is helpful to focus one's prayers on Christ, suffering and crucified, and it is recommended that one prays before a crucifix. As you seek discernment and consolation during this difficult time, the following prayers are a source of help and strength.

Psalm 6:2–3

Be merciful to me, Lord, for I am faint;
O Lord, heal me, for my bones are in agony.
My soul is in anguish.
How long, O Lord, how long?

Psalm 22:14–15

I am poured out like water,
    and all my bones are out of joint.
My heart has turned to wax;
    it has melted away within me.
My strength is dried up like a potsherd
        and my tongue sticks to the roof of my
            mouth;
you lay me in the dust of death.

The story of the sufferings of Job, the just man of the Old Testament offers an excellent meditation in times of suffering. Note especially Job's complaints in chapter 30; perhaps Jesus reflected on Job's plight. Complaining to God is indeed a prayer, one which God accepts and listens to.

Job 30:16–21, 27–31
(Job's complaint)

And now my life ebbs away;
    days of suffering rip me.
Night pierces my bones;

my gnawing pains never rest.
In his great power God becomes like clothing
    to me;
    he binds me like the neck of my garment.
He throws me into the mud,
    and I am reduced to dust and ashes.
I cry out to you, O God, but you do not
    answer;
I stand up, but you merely look at me.
You turn on me ruthlessly;
    with the might of your hand you
    attack me.
The churning inside me never stops;
    days of suffering confront me.
I go about blackened, but not by the sun;
I stand up in the assembly and cry for help.
I have become a brother of jackals,
    a companion of owls.
My skin grows black and peels;
    my body burns with fever.
My harp is tuned to mourning,
    and my flute to the sound of wailing.

Job: 38:2–5; 40:2

(God's response)

Who is this that darkens my counsel
with words without knowledge?
Brace yourself like a man;
I will question you;
    and you shall answer me.
Where were you when I laid the earth's
    foundation?
Tell me, if you understand.
Will the one who contends with the Almighty
    correct him?
Let him who accuses God answer him!

The New Testament offers numerous passages for prayer and meditation. The words of the Lord's Prayer are most powerful because Jesus himself taught it. During times of sickness the most effective part of the prayer is the abandoning of ourselves to God's will: "Thy will be done" (cf. Mt 6:10).

Christ's obedience to the Father is highlighted in the Agony in the Garden, "Father, if you are willing, take this cup from me; yet not my will, but yours be done" (Lk 22:42).

The angel ministered to Jesus after his heartfelt prayer to the Father; this consolation is yours too! "An angel from heaven appeared to him and strengthened him" (Lk 22:43).

And finally, on the cross, Jesus uttered his words of total submission to God: "Father, into your hands I commit my spirit" (Lk 23:46).

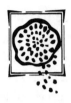

Glossary

Comfort Measures Only—ordinary means of food, hydration, cleanliness, palliative care.

Extraordinary (disproportionate) Means—specific means for a specific patient that would involve grave hardships to that patient, e.g. too painful, too costly, too unusual. A person who decides to forego treatment or have it withdrawn is not necessarily choosing death. Rather, he or she chooses life without the burden of disproportionate medical intervention, accepting the inevitability of the dying process.

However, if the patient is in a Persistent Vegetative State (PVS), this illness is not terminal; in this situation it would be morally wrong to discontinue nutrition and hydration, for this constitutes normal care. If removed, this is euthanasia by omission rather that positive lethal action. It introduces a new cause of death, namely malnutrition and/or dehydration.

Health Care Proxy (Durable Power of Attorney)—someone whom you authorize to act on your behalf when you become unable to communicate your informed consent because of illness or injury.

Living Will—a document that provides instructions regarding your medical treatment care when you are unable to communicate your informed consent because of illness or injury.

Ordinary (proportionate) Means—those means whose use does not entail grave hardship to the patient, e.g., readily available, of true benefit, and not burdensome: physically in regard to the patient, psychologically in regard to the patient, economically in regard to the family.

Palliative Care—all pain can be managed; when used with a skillful respect for the patient's perception of his or her condition, current techniques of pain control can provide great relief of most physical pain associated with terminal illness.

Physicians are morally and professionally obligated to treat pain adequately. Further, it is morally acceptable for physicians to treat pain adequately even when, in exceptional cases, the treatment indirectly hastens death. Such treatment differs from assisted suicide in that the purpose of the treatment is to relieve pain and not to cause death.

Persistent Vegetative State (PVS)—persons in a state of deep unconsciousness who are apparently unable to engage in such activities as thinking, willing or communicating because of impairment of the upper part of the brain. The brain stem, which controls such involuntary functions as breathing, blinking, cycles of waking and sleeping etc., still functions. Although persons in this state are unlikely to recover consciousness, they are in no immediate danger of death so long as they are nourished.

There is also a real question as to some physicians' ability to determine whether or not a significant number of patients diagnosed as being in persistent vegetative states are conscious. In some cases there are graded and indeterminate states of consciousness.

The term *persistent* vegetative state is preferred to the more common *permanent* vegetative state. The finality which permanent connotes is misleading since some diagnosed as such have regained consciousness.

Time of Death—it is acceptable to assume that a person is dead when the whole brain is dead, including the stem (cerebral cortex); this is the actual practice in Catholic hospitals. There are two types of brain death: partial=neo-cortex (cognitive function) and total=neo-cortex and brain stem (controls involuntary bodily activities, i.e. cessation of cardiopulmonary function).

Withdrawal of Treatment—if death is imminent, nourishment may add briefly to a life span by simply prolonging death without actually preserving life, e.g. in the case of the end stage of terminal illness. It is permitted to withdraw even nutrition, hydration, artificial respiration and dialysis from a patient, if supplying these are futile or excessively burdensome.

It is important to recognize what distinguishes this teaching from assisted suicide. In foregoing or withdrawing burdensome treatment or technological assistance, the disease causes the death; in assisted suicide, people cause the death.

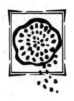

Suggested Reading

Church Documents

Archdiocese of Atlanta. 1989. "Georgia Man Asks to Turn Off Life Supporting Ventilator." *Origins* vol. 19: n. 17, pp. 273–279.

Bishops of Pennsylvania. 1992. "Nutrition and Hydration: Moral Considerations." *Origins* vol. 21: n. 34, pp. 541–553.

John Paul II. 1988. "Building a Culture of Life" (*ad limina* address to bishops from California, Hawaii, and Nevada). *Origins* vol. 28: n. 18, pp. 314–316.

John Paul II. 1995. *The Gospel of Life,* Evangelium Vitae. Boston: Pauline Books & Media.

U.S. Bishops' Pro Life Committee. 1992. "Nutrition and Hydration: Moral and Pastoral Reflections." *Origins* vol. 21: n. 44, pp. 705–712.

National Conference of Catholic Bishops. 1994. "Ethical and Religious Directives for Catholic Health Care Services." *Origins* vol. 24: n. 27, pp. 450–464.

Pontifical Council for Pastoral Assistance. 1995. *Charter for Health Care Workers*. Boston: Pauline Books & Media.

Other References

Byrne, P.A., et. al. "Life, Life Support, and Death Principles, Guidelines, Policies and Procedures for Making Decisions that Respect Life." *The Linacre Quarterly* vol. 64: n. 4, pp. 3–31.

Diamond, E.F. 1998. "Brain-Based Determination of Death Revisited." *The Linacre Quarterly* vol. 65: n. 4, pp. 71–80.

Howespian, A.A. 1998. "In Defense of Whole Brain Definitions of Death." *The Linacre Quarterly* vol. 65: n. 4, pp. 39–61.

May, W.E. 1998. "The Feeding Tube and the Vegetative State." *Ethics and Medics* vol. 23: n. 12, pp. 1–2.

May, W.E. 1999. "Tube Feeding and the Vegetative State." *Ethics and Medics* vol. 24: n. 1, pp. 1–3.

Seifert, W.N., Urbine, W.F., Orsi, M.P. 1996. *Proclaiming the Gospel of Life: A Summary and Commentary on The Gospel of Life.* Boston: Pauline Books & Media.

BOOKS & MEDIA

The Daughters of St. Paul operate book and media centers at the following addresses. Visit, call or write the one nearest you today, or find us on the World Wide Web, www.pauline.org

California
3908 Sepulveda Blvd., Culver City, CA 90230; 310-397-8676
5945 Balboa Ave., San Diego, CA 92111; 858-565-9181
46 Geary Street, San Francisco, CA 94108; 415-781-5180

Florida
145 S.W. 107th Ave., Miami, FL 33174; 305-559-6715

Hawaii
1143 Bishop Street, Honolulu, HI 96813; 808-521-2731

Neighbor Islands call: 800-259-8463

Illinois
172 North Michigan Ave., Chicago, IL 60601; 312-346-4228

Louisiana
4403 Veterans Memorial Blvd., Metairie, LA 70006; 504-887-7631

Massachusetts
Rte. 1, 885 Providence Hwy., Dedham, MA 02026; 781-326-5385

Missouri
9804 Watson Rd., St. Louis, MO 63126; 314-965-3512

New Jersey
561 U.S. Route 1, Wick Plaza, Edison, NJ 08817; 732-572-1200

New York
150 East 52nd Street, New York, NY 10022; 212-754-1110
78 Fort Place, Staten Island, NY 10301; 718-447-5071

Ohio
2105 Ontario Street, Cleveland, OH 44115; 216-621-9427

Pennsylvania
9171-A Roosevelt Blvd., Philadelphia, PA 19114; 215-676-9494

South Carolina
243 King Street, Charleston, SC 29401; 843-577-0175

Tennessee
4811 Poplar Ave., Memphis, TN 38117; 901-761-2987

Texas
114 Main Plaza, San Antonio, TX 78205; 210-224-8101

Virginia
1025 King Street, Alexandria, VA 22314; 703-549-3806

Canada
3022 Dufferin Street, Toronto, Ontario, Canada M6B 3T5; 416-781-9131
1155 Yonge Street, Toronto, Ontario, Canada M4T 1W2; 416-934-3440

¡También somos su fuente para libros, videos y música en español!